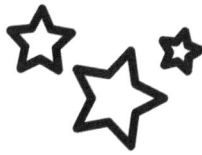

Congratulations

Congratulations on making the decision to change your life.

Changing your diet can have many benefits, including:
• Weight loss and maintenance
• Prevention and reversal of heart disease
• Prevention and reversal of diabetes
• Prevention of some types of cancer.

This lifestyle diet change though, has to be maintained over the long term. This is why this journal is for a year and not for 90 days like many of the journals are.

This journal is different to most diet journals.

This journal was written predominately for those choosing to adopt a whole-foods plant-based diet. It therefore does not count calories nor does it have sections for speed foods or treats.

This journal has one section each day for food, as if you are having the same breakfast most days, there may not be need to write that every day. Also, you do not need to write out individual ingredients. This book, therefore acts more as a journal to track your progress than it does a food diary.

On the initial page and the progress pages there are five blank lines. These are for you to monitor any medical markers that you are following, such as: cholesterol, HbA1c (diabetes), Lp-PLA2 (indicator of plaque build-up) or anything relevant to you.

This book is suitable if you are starting out on your journey or you are continuing to monitor a journey you started some time ago.

All the best in your journey.

Your food can promote health or disease – the choice is yours.

Initial

Physical Measurements:

Weight: _____ BMI: _____

Waist: _____ Thigh: _____

Hips: _____ Calf: _____

Chest: _____ Arm: _____

Any other measurements:

My Goal:

My Why:

Week Beginning: _____

Monday

🍎 Food:

_____

_____

_____

_____

Mood: 😄 😐 ☹️

✏️ Notes:

Water 💧
_____

Exercise 🏋️
_____

Sleep ⏱️
_____

Tuesday

🍎 Food:

_____

_____

_____

_____

Mood: 😄 😐 ☹️

✏️ Notes:

Water 💧
_____

Exercise 🏋️
_____

Sleep ⏱️
_____

Wednesday

🍎 Food:

_____

_____

_____

_____

Mood: 😄 😐 ☹️

✏️ Notes:

Water 💧
_____

Exercise 🏋️
_____

Sleep ⏱️
_____

Thursday

🍎 Food:

_____

_____

_____

_____

Mood: 😄 😐 ☹️

✏️ Notes:

Water 💧
_____

Exercise 🏋️
_____

Sleep ⏱️
_____

"Only I can change my life. No one can do it but me." Carol Burnett

Friday

🍎 Food:

_____
_____
_____
_____

Mood: 😄 😐 ☹️

✎ Notes:

Water 💧
_____

Exercise 🏋️
_____

Sleep ⏱️
_____

Saturday

🍎 Food:

_____
_____
_____
_____

Mood: 😄 😐 ☹️

✎ Notes:

Water 💧
_____

Exercise 🏋️
_____

Sleep ⏱️
_____

Sunday

🍎 Food:

_____
_____
_____
_____

Mood: 😄 😐 ☹️

✎ Notes:

Water 💧
_____

Exercise 🏋️
_____

Sleep ⏱️
_____

Week Overview

General mood: 😄 😐 ☹️

⚖️ Weight: _____

▭ Waist: _____

What went well:

_____
_____

To improve:

_____
_____

Week Beginning: _____

Monday

🍎 Food:

_____
_____
_____
_____

Mood: 😄 😐 ☹️

✎ Notes:

Water 💧
_____
Exercise 🏋️
_____
Sleep ⏱️
_____

Tuesday

🍎 Food:

_____
_____
_____
_____

Mood: 😄 😐 ☹️

✎ Notes:

Water 💧
_____
Exercise 🏋️
_____
Sleep ⏱️
_____

Wednesday

🍎 Food:

_____
_____
_____
_____

Mood: 😄 😐 ☹️

✎ Notes:

Water 💧
_____
Exercise 🏋️
_____
Sleep ⏱️
_____

Thursday

🍎 Food:

_____
_____
_____
_____

Mood: 😄 😐 ☹️

✎ Notes:

Water 💧
_____
Exercise 🏋️
_____
Sleep ⏱️
_____

"The starting point of all achievement is desire." Napoleon Hill

Friday

🍎 Food:

_____

_____

_____

_____

Mood: 😄 😐 ☹️

✏️ Notes:

Water 💧

_____

Exercise 🏋️

_____

Sleep ⏱️

_____

Saturday

🍎 Food:

_____

_____

_____

_____

Mood: 😄 😐 ☹️

✏️ Notes:

Water 💧

_____

Exercise 🏋️

_____

Sleep ⏱️

_____

Sunday

🍎 Food:

_____

_____

_____

_____

Mood: 😄 😐 ☹️

✏️ Notes:

Water 💧

_____

Exercise 🏋️

_____

Sleep ⏱️

_____

Week Overview

General mood: 😄 😐 ☹️

⚖️ Weight: _____

➖ Waist: _____

What went well:

_____

_____

To improve:

_____

_____

Week Beginning: _____

Monday

🍎 Food:
_____
_____
_____
_____

Mood: 😄 😐 ☹️

✒️ Notes:

Water 💧
_____
Exercise 🏋️
_____
Sleep ⏱️
_____

Tuesday

🍎 Food:
_____
_____
_____
_____

Mood: 😄 😐 ☹️

✒️ Notes:

Water 💧
_____
Exercise 🏋️
_____
Sleep ⏱️
_____

Wednesday

🍎 Food:
_____
_____
_____
_____

Mood: 😄 😐 ☹️

✒️ Notes:

Water 💧
_____
Exercise 🏋️
_____
Sleep ⏱️
_____

Thursday

🍎 Food:
_____
_____
_____
_____

Mood: 😄 😐 ☹️

✒️ Notes:

Water 💧
_____
Exercise 🏋️
_____
Sleep ⏱️
_____

"Failure will never overtake me if my determination to succeed is strong enough."
Og Mandino

Friday

🍎 Food:

_____
_____
_____
_____

Mood: 😄 😐 ☹️

✏️ Notes:

Water 💧
_____

Exercise 🏋️
_____

Sleep ⏱️
_____

Saturday

🍎 Food:

_____
_____
_____
_____

Mood: 😄 😐 ☹️

✏️ Notes:

Water 💧
_____

Exercise 🏋️
_____

Sleep ⏱️
_____

Sunday

🍎 Food:

_____
_____
_____
_____

Mood: 😄 😐 ☹️

✏️ Notes:

Water 💧
_____

Exercise 🏋️
_____

Sleep ⏱️
_____

Week Overview

General mood: 😄 😐 ☹️

⚖️ Weight: _____

➖ Waist: _____

What went well:

_____
_____

To improve:

_____
_____

Week Beginning: _____

Monday

🍎 Food:
_____
_____
_____
_____

Mood: 😄 😐 ☹️   Water 💧
_____
✏️ Notes:
Exercise 🏋️
_____
Sleep ⏱️
_____

Tuesday

🍎 Food:
_____
_____
_____
_____

Mood: 😄 😐 ☹️   Water 💧
_____
✏️ Notes:
Exercise 🏋️
_____
Sleep ⏱️
_____

Wednesday

🍎 Food:
_____
_____
_____
_____

Mood: 😄 😐 ☹️   Water 💧
_____
✏️ Notes:
Exercise 🏋️
_____
Sleep ⏱️
_____

Thursday

🍎 Food:
_____
_____
_____
_____

Mood: 😄 😐 ☹️   Water 💧
_____
✏️ Notes:
Exercise 🏋️
_____
Sleep ⏱️
_____

"Your future health can be predicted by the nutrient density of your diet." Joel Fuhrman

Friday

🍎 Food:

_____

_____

_____

_____

Mood: 😄 😐 ☹️

✎ Notes:

Water 💧

_____

Exercise 🏋️

_____

Sleep ⏱️

_____

Saturday

🍎 Food:

_____

_____

_____

_____

Mood: 😄 😐 ☹️

✎ Notes:

Water 💧

_____

Exercise 🏋️

_____

Sleep ⏱️

_____

Sunday

🍎 Food:

_____

_____

_____

_____

Mood: 😄 😐 ☹️

✎ Notes:

Water 💧

_____

Exercise 🏋️

_____

Sleep ⏱️

_____

Week Overview

General mood: 😄 😐 ☹️

⚖️ Weight: _____

➖ Waist: _____

What went well:

_____

_____

To improve:

_____

_____

Week Beginning: _____

Monday

🍎 Food:

_____
_____
_____
_____

Mood: 😄 😐 ☹️   Water 💧
_____

✏️ Notes: Exercise 🏋️
_____

Sleep ⏱️
_____

Tuesday

🍎 Food:

_____
_____
_____
_____

Mood: 😄 😐 ☹️   Water 💧
_____

✏️ Notes: Exercise 🏋️
_____

Sleep ⏱️
_____

Wednesday

🍎 Food:

_____
_____
_____
_____

Mood: 😄 😐 ☹️   Water 💧
_____

✏️ Notes: Exercise 🏋️
_____

Sleep ⏱️
_____

Thursday

🍎 Food:

_____
_____
_____
_____

Mood: 😄 😐 ☹️   Water 💧
_____

✏️ Notes: Exercise 🏋️
_____

Sleep ⏱️
_____

"You have to be at your strongest when you're feeling at your weakest."

Friday

🍎 Food:

_____
_____
_____
_____

Mood: 😄 😐 ☹️

✏️ Notes:

Water 💧
_____

Exercise 🏋️
_____

Sleep ⏱️
_____

Saturday

🍎 Food:

_____
_____
_____
_____

Mood: 😄 😐 ☹️

✏️ Notes:

Water 💧
_____

Exercise 🏋️
_____

Sleep ⏱️
_____

Sunday

🍎 Food:

_____
_____
_____
_____

Mood: 😄 😐 ☹️

✏️ Notes:

Water 💧
_____

Exercise 🏋️
_____

Sleep ⏱️
_____

Week Overview

General mood: 😄 😐 ☹️

⚖️ Weight: _____

➖ Waist: _____

What went well:

To improve:

Week Beginning: _____

Monday

🍎 Food:

_____
_____
_____
_____

Mood: 😄 😐 ☹️   Water 💧
_____

✏️ Notes:

Exercise 🏋️
_____

Sleep ⏱️
_____

Tuesday

🍎 Food:

_____
_____
_____
_____

Mood: 😄 😐 ☹️   Water 💧
_____

✏️ Notes:

Exercise 🏋️
_____

Sleep ⏱️
_____

Wednesday

🍎 Food:

_____
_____
_____
_____

Mood: 😄 😐 ☹️   Water 💧
_____

✏️ Notes:

Exercise 🏋️
_____

Sleep ⏱️
_____

Thursday

🍎 Food:

_____
_____
_____
_____

Mood: 😄 😐 ☹️   Water 💧
_____

✏️ Notes:

Exercise 🏋️
_____

Sleep ⏱️
_____

"A healthy diet has a direct link to increased cognitive function and memory skills, decreased absenteeism from school, and improved mood." Matt Cartwright

Friday

🍎 Food:

_____

_____

_____

_____

Mood: 😄 😐 ☹️

✏️ Notes:

Water 💧

_____

Exercise 🏋️

_____

Sleep ⏱️

_____

Saturday

🍎 Food:

_____

_____

_____

_____

Mood: 😄 😐 ☹️

✏️ Notes:

Water 💧

_____

Exercise 🏋️

_____

Sleep ⏱️

_____

Sunday

🍎 Food:

_____

_____

_____

_____

Mood: 😄 😐 ☹️

✏️ Notes:

Water 💧

_____

Exercise 🏋️

_____

Sleep ⏱️

_____

Week Overview

General mood: 😄 😐 ☹️

⚖️ Weight: _____

➖ Waist: _____

What went well:

_____

_____

To improve:

_____

Week Beginning: _____

Monday

🍎 Food:

_____
_____
_____
_____

Mood: 😄 😐 ☹️   Water 💧

✏️ Notes: _____

Exercise 🏋️
_____

Sleep ⏱️
_____

Tuesday

🍎 Food:

_____
_____
_____
_____

Mood: 😄 😐 ☹️   Water 💧

✏️ Notes: _____

Exercise 🏋️
_____

Sleep ⏱️
_____

Wednesday

🍎 Food:

_____
_____
_____
_____

Mood: 😄 😐 ☹️   Water 💧

✏️ Notes: _____

Exercise 🏋️
_____

Sleep ⏱️
_____

Thursday

🍎 Food:

_____
_____
_____
_____

Mood: 😄 😐 ☹️   Water 💧

✏️ Notes: _____

Exercise 🏋️
_____

Sleep ⏱️
_____

"Focus on your goal. Don't look in any direction but ahead."

Friday

🍎 Food:

_____

_____

_____

_____

Mood: 😄 😐 ☹️

✏️ Notes:

Water 💧

_____

Exercise 🏋️

_____

Sleep ⏱️

_____

Saturday

🍎 Food:

_____

_____

_____

_____

Mood: 😄 😐 ☹️

✏️ Notes:

Water 💧

_____

Exercise 🏋️

_____

Sleep ⏱️

_____

Sunday

🍎 Food:

_____

_____

_____

_____

Mood: 😄 😐 ☹️

✏️ Notes:

Water 💧

_____

Exercise 🏋️

_____

Sleep ⏱️

_____

Week Overview

General mood: 😄 😐 ☹️

⚖️ Weight: _____

➖ Waist: _____

What went well:

_____

_____

To improve:

_____

Week Beginning: _____

Monday

🍎 Food:

_____

_____

_____

_____

Mood: 😄 😐 ☹️   Water 💧 _____

✒️ Notes: Exercise 🏋️ _____

                    Sleep ⏱️ _____

Tuesday

🍎 Food:

_____

_____

_____

_____

Mood: 😄 😐 ☹️   Water 💧 _____

✒️ Notes: Exercise 🏋️ _____

                    Sleep ⏱️ _____

Wednesday

🍎 Food:

_____

_____

_____

_____

Mood: 😄 😐 ☹️   Water 💧 _____

✒️ Notes: Exercise 🏋️ _____

                    Sleep ⏱️ _____

Thursday

🍎 Food:

_____

_____

_____

_____

Mood: 😄 😐 ☹️   Water 💧 _____

✒️ Notes: Exercise 🏋️ _____

                    Sleep ⏱️ _____

"A balanced diet may be the best medicine."   Alton Brown

Friday

🍎 Food:

_____

_____

_____

_____

Mood: 😄 😐 😞   Water 💧

✏️ Notes: _____

Exercise 🏋️

_____

Sleep ⏱️

_____

Saturday

🍎 Food:

_____

_____

_____

_____

Mood: 😄 😐 😞   Water 💧

✏️ Notes: _____

Exercise 🏋️

_____

Sleep ⏱️

_____

Sunday

🍎 Food:

_____

_____

_____

_____

Mood: 😄 😐 😞   Water 💧

✏️ Notes: _____

Exercise 🏋️

_____

Sleep ⏱️

_____

Week Overview

General mood: 😄 😐 😞

⚖️ Weight: _____

➖ Waist: _____

What went well:

_____

_____

To improve:

_____

_____

Week Beginning: _____

Monday

🍎 Food:

_____
_____
_____
_____

Mood: 😄 😐 ☹️   Water 💧 _____

✏️ Notes:

Exercise 🏋️ _____

Sleep ⏱️ _____

Tuesday

🍎 Food:

_____
_____
_____
_____

Mood: 😄 😐 ☹️   Water 💧 _____

✏️ Notes:

Exercise 🏋️ _____

Sleep ⏱️ _____

Wednesday

🍎 Food:

_____
_____
_____
_____

Mood: 😄 😐 ☹️   Water 💧 _____

✏️ Notes:

Exercise 🏋️ _____

Sleep ⏱️ _____

Thursday

🍎 Food:

_____
_____
_____
_____

Mood: 😄 😐 ☹️   Water 💧 _____

✏️ Notes:

Exercise 🏋️ _____

Sleep ⏱️ _____

"Whatever your problem is, the answer is not in the fridge." Karen Salmansohn

Friday

🍎 Food:

_____
_____
_____
_____

Mood: 😄 😐 ☹️

✍️ Notes:

Water 💧
_____

Exercise 🏋️
_____

Sleep ⏱️
_____

Saturday

🍎 Food:

_____
_____
_____
_____

Mood: 😄 😐 ☹️

✍️ Notes:

Water 💧
_____

Exercise 🏋️
_____

Sleep ⏱️
_____

Sunday

🍎 Food:

_____
_____
_____
_____

Mood: 😄 😐 ☹️

✍️ Notes:

Water 💧
_____

Exercise 🏋️
_____

Sleep ⏱️
_____

Week Overview

General mood: 😄 😐 ☹️

⚖️ Weight: _____

➖ Waist: _____

What went well:

_____
_____

To improve:

_____

Week Beginning: _____

Monday

🍎 Food:

_____
_____
_____
_____

Mood: 😄 😐 ☹️   Water 💧

✏️ Notes: _____

Exercise 🏋️   _____

Sleep ⏱️   _____

Tuesday

🍎 Food:

_____
_____
_____
_____

Mood: 😄 😐 ☹️   Water 💧

✏️ Notes: _____

Exercise 🏋️   _____

Sleep ⏱️   _____

Wednesday

🍎 Food:

_____
_____
_____
_____

Mood: 😄 😐 ☹️   Water 💧

✏️ Notes: _____

Exercise 🏋️   _____

Sleep ⏱️   _____

Thursday

🍎 Food:

_____
_____
_____
_____

Mood: 😄 😐 ☹️   Water 💧

✏️ Notes: _____

Exercise 🏋️   _____

Sleep ⏱️   _____

"What you do today can improve all your tomorrows." Ralph Marston

Friday

🍎 Food:

_____
_____
_____
_____

Mood: 😄 😐 ☹️

✎ Notes:

Water 💧
_____

Exercise 🏋️
_____

Sleep ⏱️
_____

Saturday

🍎 Food:

_____
_____
_____
_____

Mood: 😄 😐 ☹️

✎ Notes:

Water 💧
_____

Exercise 🏋️
_____

Sleep ⏱️
_____

Sunday

🍎 Food:

_____
_____
_____
_____

Mood: 😄 😐 ☹️

✎ Notes:

Water 💧
_____

Exercise 🏋️
_____

Sleep ⏱️
_____

Week Overview

General mood: 😄 😐 ☹️

⚖️ Weight: _____

➖ Waist: _____

What went well:
_____
_____

To improve:
_____

Week Beginning: _____

Monday

🍎 Food:

_____

_____

_____

_____

Mood: 😄 😐 ☹️

✏️ Notes:

Water 💧
_____

Exercise 🏋️
_____

Sleep ⏱️
_____

Tuesday

🍎 Food:

_____

_____

_____

_____

Mood: 😄 😐 ☹️

✏️ Notes:

Water 💧
_____

Exercise 🏋️
_____

Sleep ⏱️
_____

Wednesday

🍎 Food:

_____

_____

_____

_____

Mood: 😄 😐 ☹️

✏️ Notes:

Water 💧
_____

Exercise 🏋️
_____

Sleep ⏱️
_____

Thursday

🍎 Food:

_____

_____

_____

_____

Mood: 😄 😐 ☹️

✏️ Notes:

Water 💧
_____

Exercise 🏋️
_____

Sleep ⏱️
_____

"It always seems impossible until it's done." Nelson Mandela

Friday

🍎 Food:

_____

_____

_____

_____

Mood: 😄 😐 ☹️

✏️ Notes:

Water 💧

_____

Exercise 🏋️

_____

Sleep ⏱️

_____

Saturday

🍎 Food:

_____

_____

_____

_____

Mood: 😄 😐 ☹️

✏️ Notes:

Water 💧

_____

Exercise 🏋️

_____

Sleep ⏱️

_____

Sunday

🍎 Food:

_____

_____

_____

_____

Mood: 😄 😐 ☹️

✏️ Notes:

Water 💧

_____

Exercise 🏋️

_____

Sleep ⏱️

_____

Week Overview

General mood: 😄 😐 ☹️

⚖️ Weight: _____

▬ Waist: _____

What went well:

_____

_____

To improve:

_____

_____

Week Beginning: _____

Monday

🍎 Food:

_____
_____
_____

Mood: 😄 😐 ☹️   Water 💧
🖊 Notes:
_____
Exercise 🏋️
_____
Sleep ⏱
_____

Tuesday

🍎 Food:

_____
_____
_____

Mood: 😄 😐 ☹️   Water 💧
🖊 Notes:
_____
Exercise 🏋️
_____
Sleep ⏱
_____

Wednesday

🍎 Food:

_____
_____
_____

Mood: 😄 😐 ☹️   Water 💧
🖊 Notes:
_____
Exercise 🏋️
_____
Sleep ⏱
_____

Thursday

🍎 Food:

_____
_____
_____

Mood: 😄 😐 ☹️   Water 💧
🖊 Notes:
_____
Exercise 🏋️
_____
Sleep ⏱
_____

"Quality is not an act, it is a habit." Aristotle

Friday

🍎 Food:

_____
_____
_____
_____

Mood: 😄 😐 ☹️

✏️ Notes:

Water 💧
_____

Exercise 🏋️
_____

Sleep ⏱️
_____

Saturday

🍎 Food:

_____
_____
_____
_____

Mood: 😄 😐 ☹️

✏️ Notes:

Water 💧
_____

Exercise 🏋️
_____

Sleep ⏱️
_____

Sunday

🍎 Food:

_____
_____
_____
_____

Mood: 😄 😐 ☹️

✏️ Notes:

Water 💧
_____

Exercise 🏋️
_____

Sleep ⏱️
_____

Week Overview

General mood: 😄 😐 ☹️

⚖️ Weight: _____

➖ Waist: _____

What went well:

To improve:

Week Beginning: _____

Monday

🍎 Food:

_____
_____
_____
_____

Mood: 😄 😐 ☹️

✏️ Notes:

Water 💧 _____

Exercise 🏋️ _____

Sleep ⏱️ _____

Tuesday

🍎 Food:

_____
_____
_____
_____

Mood: 😄 😐 ☹️

✏️ Notes:

Water 💧 _____

Exercise 🏋️ _____

Sleep ⏱️ _____

Wednesday

🍎 Food:

_____
_____
_____
_____

Mood: 😄 😐 ☹️

✏️ Notes:

Water 💧 _____

Exercise 🏋️ _____

Sleep ⏱️ _____

Thursday

🍎 Food:

_____
_____
_____
_____

Mood: 😄 😐 ☹️

✏️ Notes:

Water 💧 _____

Exercise 🏋️ _____

Sleep ⏱️ _____

"Without hard work, nothing grows but weeds." Gordon B. Hinckley

Friday

🍎 Food:

_____
_____
_____
_____

Mood: 😄 😐 ☹️

✎ Notes:

Water 💧
_____

Exercise 🏋️
_____

Sleep ⏱️
_____

Saturday

🍎 Food:

_____
_____
_____
_____

Mood: 😄 😐 ☹️

✎ Notes:

Water 💧
_____

Exercise 🏋️
_____

Sleep ⏱️
_____

Sunday

🍎 Food:

_____
_____
_____
_____

Mood: 😄 😐 ☹️

✎ Notes:

Water 💧
_____

Exercise 🏋️
_____

Sleep ⏱️
_____

Week Overview

General mood: 😄 😐 ☹️

⚖️ Weight: _____

➖ Waist: _____

What went well:

_____
_____

To improve:

_____
_____

Yes,
I can

Three Monthly Review

Well done you have completed three months.

Physical Measurements:

Weight:	Change in weight:
Waist:	Change in waist:
Hips:	Change in hips:
Thigh:	Change in thigh:

Any other measurements:

	Change:
	Change:
	Change:
	Change:

Best thing about the last three months:

What I need to improve:

Main goal for next three months:

Week Beginning: _____

Monday

🍎 Food:

_____
_____
_____

Mood: 😄 😐 ☹️   Water 💧 _____

✏️ Notes: Exercise 🏋️ _____

                                   Sleep ⏱️ _____

Tuesday

🍎 Food:

_____
_____
_____

Mood: 😄 😐 ☹️   Water 💧 _____

✏️ Notes: Exercise 🏋️ _____

                                   Sleep ⏱️ _____

Wednesday

🍎 Food:

_____
_____
_____

Mood: 😄 😐 ☹️   Water 💧 _____

✏️ Notes: Exercise 🏋️ _____

                                   Sleep ⏱️ _____

Thursday

🍎 Food:

_____
_____
_____

Mood: 😄 😐 ☹️   Water 💧 _____

✏️ Notes: Exercise 🏋️ _____

                                   Sleep ⏱️ _____

"The groundwork of all happiness is health." Leigh Hunt

Friday

🍎 Food:

_____
_____
_____
_____

Mood: 😄 😐 ☹️

✏️ Notes:

Water 💧
_____

Exercise 🏋️
_____

Sleep ⏱️
_____

Saturday

🍎 Food:

_____
_____
_____
_____

Mood: 😄 😐 ☹️

✏️ Notes:

Water 💧
_____

Exercise 🏋️
_____

Sleep ⏱️
_____

Sunday

🍎 Food:

_____
_____
_____
_____

Mood: 😄 😐 ☹️

✏️ Notes:

Water 💧
_____

Exercise 🏋️
_____

Sleep ⏱️
_____

Week Overview

General mood: 😄 😐 ☹️

⚖️ Weight: _____

➖ Waist: _____

What went well:

To improve:

Week Beginning: _____

Monday

🍎 Food:

_____

_____

_____

_____

Mood: 😄 😐 ☹️   Water 💧

✏️ Notes: _____

                   Exercise 🏋️

                   _____

                   Sleep ⏱️

                   _____

Tuesday

🍎 Food:

_____

_____

_____

_____

Mood: 😄 😐 ☹️   Water 💧

✏️ Notes: _____

                   Exercise 🏋️

                   _____

                   Sleep ⏱️

                   _____

Wednesday

🍎 Food:

_____

_____

_____

_____

Mood: 😄 😐 ☹️   Water 💧

✏️ Notes: _____

                   Exercise 🏋️

                   _____

                   Sleep ⏱️

                   _____

Thursday

🍎 Food:

_____

_____

_____

_____

Mood: 😄 😐 ☹️   Water 💧

✏️ Notes: _____

                   Exercise 🏋️

                   _____

                   Sleep ⏱️

                   _____

"Never give up. Great things take time. Be patient."

Friday

🍎 Food:

_____
_____
_____
_____

Mood: 😄 😐 🙁   Water 💧
✏️ Notes: _____

                                 Exercise 🏋️
                                 _____

                                 Sleep ⏱️
                                 _____

Saturday

🍎 Food:

_____
_____
_____
_____

Mood: 😄 😐 🙁   Water 💧
✏️ Notes: _____

                                 Exercise 🏋️
                                 _____

                                 Sleep ⏱️
                                 _____

Sunday

🍎 Food:

_____
_____
_____
_____

Mood: 😄 😐 🙁   Water 💧
✏️ Notes: _____

                                 Exercise 🏋️
                                 _____

                                 Sleep ⏱️
                                 _____

Week Overview

General mood: 😄 😐 🙁

⚖️ Weight: _____

➖ Waist: _____

What went well:

_____
_____

To improve:

_____
_____

Week Beginning: _____

Monday

🍎 Food:

_____
_____
_____
_____

Mood: 😄 😐 ☹️

✏️ Notes:

Water 💧
_____
Exercise 🏋️
_____
Sleep ⏱️

Tuesday

🍎 Food:

_____
_____
_____
_____

Mood: 😄 😐 ☹️

✏️ Notes:

Water 💧
_____
Exercise 🏋️
_____
Sleep ⏱️

Wednesday

🍎 Food:

_____
_____
_____
_____

Mood: 😄 😐 ☹️

✏️ Notes:

Water 💧
_____
Exercise 🏋️
_____
Sleep ⏱️

Thursday

🍎 Food:

_____
_____
_____
_____

Mood: 😄 😐 ☹️

✏️ Notes:

Water 💧
_____
Exercise 🏋️
_____
Sleep ⏱️

"If you feel like giving up, just look back at how far you have already come."

Friday

🍎 Food:

_____

_____

_____

_____

Mood: 😄 😐 ☹️

✏️ Notes:

Water 💧

_____

Exercise 🏋️

_____

Sleep ⏱️

_____

Saturday

🍎 Food:

_____

_____

_____

_____

Mood: 😄 😐 ☹️

✏️ Notes:

Water 💧

_____

Exercise 🏋️

_____

Sleep ⏱️

_____

Sunday

🍎 Food:

_____

_____

_____

_____

Mood: 😄 😐 ☹️

✏️ Notes:

Water 💧

_____

Exercise 🏋️

_____

Sleep ⏱️

_____

Week Overview

General mood: 😄 😐 ☹️

⚖️ Weight: _____

▬ Waist: _____

What went well:

_____

_____

To improve:

_____

Week Beginning: _____

Monday

🍎 Food:
_____
_____
_____

Mood: 😄 😐 ☹️   Water 💧 _____

Notes: _____

Exercise 🏋️ _____

Sleep ⏱️ _____

Tuesday

🍎 Food:
_____
_____
_____

Mood: 😄 😐 ☹️   Water 💧 _____

Notes: _____

Exercise 🏋️ _____

Sleep ⏱️ _____

Wednesday

🍎 Food:
_____
_____
_____

Mood: 😄 😐 ☹️   Water 💧 _____

Notes: _____

Exercise 🏋️ _____

Sleep ⏱️ _____

Thursday

🍎 Food:
_____
_____
_____

Mood: 😄 😐 ☹️   Water 💧 _____

Notes: _____

Exercise 🏋️ _____

Sleep ⏱️ _____

"I didn't get there by wishing for it or hoping for it, but by working for it." Estée Lauder

Friday

🍎 Food:

_____
_____
_____
_____

Mood: 😄 😐 🙁

✏️ Notes:

Water 💧
_____

Exercise 🏋️
_____

Sleep ⏱️
_____

Saturday

🍎 Food:

_____
_____
_____
_____

Mood: 😄 😐 🙁

✏️ Notes:

Water 💧
_____

Exercise 🏋️
_____

Sleep ⏱️
_____

Sunday

🍎 Food:

_____
_____
_____
_____

Mood: 😄 😐 🙁

✏️ Notes:

Water 💧
_____

Exercise 🏋️
_____

Sleep ⏱️
_____

Week Overview

General mood: 😄 😐 🙁

⚖️ Weight: _____

➖ Waist: _____

What went well:

To improve:

Week Beginning: _____

Monday

🍎 Food:

_____
_____
_____
_____

Mood: 😄 😐 ☹️

✏️ Notes:

Water 💧
_____

Exercise 🏋️
_____

Sleep ⏱️

Tuesday

🍎 Food:

_____
_____
_____
_____

Mood: 😄 😐 ☹️

✏️ Notes:

Water 💧
_____

Exercise 🏋️
_____

Sleep ⏱️

Wednesday

🍎 Food:

_____
_____
_____
_____

Mood: 😄 😐 ☹️

✏️ Notes:

Water 💧
_____

Exercise 🏋️
_____

Sleep ⏱️

Thursday

🍎 Food:

_____
_____
_____
_____

Mood: 😄 😐 ☹️

✏️ Notes:

Water 💧
_____

Exercise 🏋️
_____

Sleep ⏱️

"Grit is that 'extra something' that separates the most successful people from the rest. It's the passion, perseverance, and stamina that we must channel in order to stick with our dreams until they become a reality." Travis Bradberry

Friday

🍎 Food:

_____
_____
_____
_____

Mood: 😄 😐 😟

✏️ Notes:

Water 💧
_____

Exercise 🏋️
_____

Sleep ⏱️
_____

Saturday

🍎 Food:

_____
_____
_____
_____

Mood: 😄 😐 😟

✏️ Notes:

Water 💧
_____

Exercise 🏋️
_____

Sleep ⏱️
_____

Sunday

🍎 Food:

_____
_____
_____
_____

Mood: 😄 😐 😟

✏️ Notes:

Water 💧
_____

Exercise 🏋️
_____

Sleep ⏱️
_____

Week Overview

General mood: 😄 😐 😟

⚖️ Weight: _____

▭ Waist: _____

What went well:

_____
_____

To improve:

_____
_____

Week Beginning: _____

Monday

🍎 Food:

_____
_____
_____
_____

Mood: 😄 😐 ☹️

✎ Notes:

Water 💧
_____

Exercise 🏋️
_____

Sleep ⏱️

Tuesday

🍎 Food:

_____
_____
_____
_____

Mood: 😄 😐 ☹️

✎ Notes:

Water 💧
_____

Exercise 🏋️
_____

Sleep ⏱️

Wednesday

🍎 Food:

_____
_____
_____
_____

Mood: 😄 😐 ☹️

✎ Notes:

Water 💧
_____

Exercise 🏋️
_____

Sleep ⏱️

Thursday

🍎 Food:

_____
_____
_____
_____

Mood: 😄 😐 ☹️

✎ Notes:

Water 💧
_____

Exercise 🏋️
_____

Sleep ⏱️

"One must eat to live, not live to eat." Jean-Baptiste Poquelin

Friday

🍎 Food:

_____

_____

_____

_____

Mood: 😄 😐 ☹️

✏️ Notes:

Water 💧

_____

Exercise 🏋️

_____

Sleep ⏱️

_____

Saturday

🍎 Food:

_____

_____

_____

_____

Mood: 😄 😐 ☹️

✏️ Notes:

Water 💧

_____

Exercise 🏋️

_____

Sleep ⏱️

_____

Sunday

🍎 Food:

_____

_____

_____

_____

Mood: 😄 😐 ☹️

✏️ Notes:

Water 💧

_____

Exercise 🏋️

_____

Sleep ⏱️

_____

Week Overview

General mood: 😄 😐 ☹️

⚖️ Weight: _____

➖ Waist: _____

What went well:

_____

_____

To improve:

_____

Week Beginning: _____

Monday

🍎 Food:

_____
_____
_____
_____

Mood: 😄 😐 ☹️

✏️ Notes:

Water 💧 _____

Exercise 🏋️ _____

Sleep ⏱️ _____

Tuesday

🍎 Food:

_____
_____
_____
_____

Mood: 😄 😐 ☹️

✏️ Notes:

Water 💧 _____

Exercise 🏋️ _____

Sleep ⏱️ _____

Wednesday

🍎 Food:

_____
_____
_____
_____

Mood: 😄 😐 ☹️

✏️ Notes:

Water 💧 _____

Exercise 🏋️ _____

Sleep ⏱️ _____

Thursday

🍎 Food:

_____
_____
_____
_____

Mood: 😄 😐 ☹️

✏️ Notes:

Water 💧 _____

Exercise 🏋️ _____

Sleep ⏱️ _____

"Action is the foundational key to all success." Pablo Picasso

Friday

🍎 Food:

_____
_____
_____
_____

Mood: 😄 😐 ☹️

✏️ Notes:

Water 💧
_____

Exercise 🏋️
_____

Sleep ⏱️
_____

Saturday

🍎 Food:

_____
_____
_____
_____

Mood: 😄 😐 ☹️

✏️ Notes:

Water 💧
_____

Exercise 🏋️
_____

Sleep ⏱️
_____

Sunday

🍎 Food:

_____
_____
_____
_____

Mood: 😄 😐 ☹️

✏️ Notes:

Water 💧
_____

Exercise 🏋️
_____

Sleep ⏱️
_____

Week Overview

General mood: 😄 😐 ☹️

⚖️ Weight: _____

▬ Waist: _____

What went well:

_____
_____

To improve:

_____
_____

Week Beginning: _____

Monday

🍎 Food:

_____
_____
_____
_____

Mood: 😄 😐 ☹️

✒️ Notes:

Water 💧
_____

Exercise 🏋️
_____

Sleep ⏱️
_____

Tuesday

🍎 Food:

_____
_____
_____
_____

Mood: 😄 😐 ☹️

✒️ Notes:

Water 💧
_____

Exercise 🏋️
_____

Sleep ⏱️
_____

Wednesday

🍎 Food:

_____
_____
_____
_____

Mood: 😄 😐 ☹️

✒️ Notes:

Water 💧
_____

Exercise 🏋️
_____

Sleep ⏱️
_____

Thursday

🍎 Food:

_____
_____
_____
_____

Mood: 😄 😐 ☹️

✒️ Notes:

Water 💧
_____

Exercise 🏋️
_____

Sleep ⏱️
_____

"The difference between a successful person and others is not a lack of strength, not a lack of knowledge, but rather a lack of will." Vince Lombardi

Friday

🍎 Food:

_____
_____
_____
_____

Mood: 😄 😐 😞   Water 💧

✏️ Notes:

_____

Exercise 🏋️

_____

Sleep ⏱️

_____

Saturday

🍎 Food:

_____
_____
_____
_____

Mood: 😄 😐 😞   Water 💧

✏️ Notes:

_____

Exercise 🏋️

_____

Sleep ⏱️

_____

Sunday

🍎 Food:

_____
_____
_____
_____

Mood: 😄 😐 😞   Water 💧

✏️ Notes:

_____

Exercise 🏋️

_____

Sleep ⏱️

_____

Week Overview

General mood: 😄 😐 😞

⚖️ Weight: _____

➖ Waist: _____

What went well:

_____
_____

To improve:

_____
_____

Week Beginning: _____

Monday

🍎 Food:
_____
_____
_____
_____

Mood: 😄 😐 ☹️   Water 💧

✏️ Notes: _____

Exercise 🏋️ _____

Sleep ⏱️ _____

Tuesday

🍎 Food:
_____
_____
_____
_____

Mood: 😄 😐 ☹️   Water 💧

✏️ Notes: _____

Exercise 🏋️ _____

Sleep ⏱️ _____

Wednesday

🍎 Food:
_____
_____
_____
_____

Mood: 😄 😐 ☹️   Water 💧

✏️ Notes: _____

Exercise 🏋️ _____

Sleep ⏱️ _____

Thursday

🍎 Food:
_____
_____
_____
_____

Mood: 😄 😐 ☹️   Water 💧

✏️ Notes: _____

Exercise 🏋️ _____

Sleep ⏱️ _____

"It does not matter how slowly you go as long as you do not stop." Confucius

Friday

🍎 Food:

_____

_____

_____

_____

Mood: 😄 😐 ☹️

✏️ Notes:

Water 💧
_____

Exercise 🏋️
_____

Sleep ⏱️
_____

Saturday

🍎 Food:

_____

_____

_____

_____

Mood: 😄 😐 ☹️

✏️ Notes:

Water 💧
_____

Exercise 🏋️
_____

Sleep ⏱️
_____

Sunday

🍎 Food:

_____

_____

_____

_____

Mood: 😄 😐 ☹️

✏️ Notes:

Water 💧
_____

Exercise 🏋️
_____

Sleep ⏱️
_____

Week Overview

General mood: 😄 😐 ☹️

⚖️ Weight: _____

▬ Waist: _____

What went well:

_____

To improve:

_____

Week Beginning: _____

Monday

🍎 Food:
_____
_____
_____
_____

Mood: 😄 😐 🙁   Water 💧 _____

✏️ Notes: Exercise 🏋️ _____

Sleep ⏱️ _____

Tuesday

🍎 Food:
_____
_____
_____
_____

Mood: 😄 😐 🙁   Water 💧 _____

✏️ Notes: Exercise 🏋️ _____

Sleep ⏱️ _____

Wednesday

🍎 Food:
_____
_____
_____
_____

Mood: 😄 😐 🙁   Water 💧 _____

✏️ Notes: Exercise 🏋️ _____

Sleep ⏱️ _____

Thursday

🍎 Food:
_____
_____
_____
_____

Mood: 😄 😐 🙁   Water 💧 _____

✏️ Notes: Exercise 🏋️ _____

Sleep ⏱️ _____

"Success is the sum of small efforts, repeated day-in and day-out." Robert Collier

Friday

🍎 Food:

_____
_____
_____
_____

Mood: 😄 😐 ☹️

✎ Notes:

Water 💧
_____

Exercise 🏋️
_____

Sleep ⏱️
_____

Saturday

🍎 Food:

_____
_____
_____
_____

Mood: 😄 😐 ☹️

✎ Notes:

Water 💧
_____

Exercise 🏋️
_____

Sleep ⏱️
_____

Sunday

🍎 Food:

_____
_____
_____
_____

Mood: 😄 😐 ☹️

✎ Notes:

Water 💧
_____

Exercise 🏋️
_____

Sleep ⏱️
_____

Week Overview

General mood: 😄 😐 ☹️

⚖️ Weight: _____

➖ Waist: _____

What went well:

_____
_____

To improve:

_____

Week Beginning: _____

Monday

🍎 Food:

_____
_____
_____

Mood: 😄 😐 ☹️

✎ Notes:

Water 💧
_____

Exercise 🏋️
_____

Sleep ⏱️
_____

Tuesday

🍎 Food:

_____
_____
_____

Mood: 😄 😐 ☹️

✎ Notes:

Water 💧
_____

Exercise 🏋️
_____

Sleep ⏱️
_____

Wednesday

🍎 Food:

_____
_____
_____

Mood: 😄 😐 ☹️

✎ Notes:

Water 💧
_____

Exercise 🏋️
_____

Sleep ⏱️
_____

Thursday

🍎 Food:

_____
_____
_____

Mood: 😄 😐 ☹️

✎ Notes:

Water 💧
_____

Exercise 🏋️
_____

Sleep ⏱️
_____

"My body is getting stronger and healthier every day."

Friday

🍎 Food:

_____
_____
_____
_____

Mood: 😄 😐 ☹️

✒️ Notes:

Water 💧
_____

Exercise 🏋️
_____

Sleep ⏱️
_____

Saturday

🍎 Food:

_____
_____
_____
_____

Mood: 😄 😐 ☹️

✒️ Notes:

Water 💧
_____

Exercise 🏋️
_____

Sleep ⏱️
_____

Sunday

🍎 Food:

_____
_____
_____
_____

Mood: 😄 😐 ☹️

✒️ Notes:

Water 💧
_____

Exercise 🏋️
_____

Sleep ⏱️
_____

Week Overview

General mood: 😄 😐 ☹️

⚖️ Weight: _____

➖ Waist: _____

What went well:

_____
_____

To improve:

_____
_____

Week Beginning: _____

Monday

🍎 Food:

_____

_____

_____

Mood: 😄 😐 ☹️

✏️ Notes:

Water 💧

_____

Exercise 🏋️

_____

Sleep ⏱️

Tuesday

🍎 Food:

_____

_____

_____

Mood: 😄 😐 ☹️

✏️ Notes:

Water 💧

_____

Exercise 🏋️

_____

Sleep ⏱️

Wednesday

🍎 Food:

_____

_____

_____

Mood: 😄 😐 ☹️

✏️ Notes:

Water 💧

_____

Exercise 🏋️

_____

Sleep ⏱️

Thursday

🍎 Food:

_____

_____

_____

Mood: 😄 😐 ☹️

✏️ Notes:

Water 💧

_____

Exercise 🏋️

_____

Sleep ⏱️

"Do not be afraid of moving slowly, be afraid of standing still."

Friday

🍎 Food:

_____
_____
_____
_____

Mood: 😄 😐 🙁

✏️ Notes:

Water 💧
_____

Exercise 🏋️
_____

Sleep ⏱️
_____

Saturday

🍎 Food:

_____
_____
_____
_____

Mood: 😄 😐 🙁

✏️ Notes:

Water 💧
_____

Exercise 🏋️
_____

Sleep ⏱️
_____

Sunday

🍎 Food:

_____
_____
_____
_____

Mood: 😄 😐 🙁

✏️ Notes:

Water 💧
_____

Exercise 🏋️
_____

Sleep ⏱️
_____

Week Overview

General mood: 😄 😐 🙁

⚖️ Weight: _____

➖ Waist: _____

What went well:

_____
_____

To improve:

_____

Week Beginning: _____

Monday

🍎 Food:

_____
_____
_____
_____

Mood: 😄 😐 ☹️

✒️ Notes:

Water 💧
_____

Exercise 🏋️
_____

Sleep ⏱️
_____

Tuesday

🍎 Food:

_____
_____
_____
_____

Mood: 😄 😐 ☹️

✒️ Notes:

Water 💧
_____

Exercise 🏋️
_____

Sleep ⏱️
_____

Wednesday

🍎 Food:

_____
_____
_____
_____

Mood: 😄 😐 ☹️

✒️ Notes:

Water 💧
_____

Exercise 🏋️
_____

Sleep ⏱️
_____

Thursday

🍎 Food:

_____
_____
_____
_____

Mood: 😄 😐 ☹️

✒️ Notes:

Water 💧
_____

Exercise 🏋️
_____

Sleep ⏱️
_____

"Prove them wrong."

Friday

🍎 Food:

_____
_____
_____
_____

Mood: 😄 😐 ☹️

✎ Notes:

Water 💧
_____

Exercise 🏋️
_____

Sleep ⏱️
_____

Saturday

🍎 Food:

_____
_____
_____
_____

Mood: 😄 😐 ☹️

✎ Notes:

Water 💧
_____

Exercise 🏋️
_____

Sleep ⏱️
_____

Sunday

🍎 Food:

_____
_____
_____
_____

Mood: 😄 😐 ☹️

✎ Notes:

Water 💧
_____

Exercise 🏋️
_____

Sleep ⏱️
_____

Week Overview

General mood: 😄 😐 ☹️

⚖️ Weight: _____

▬ Waist: _____

What went well:

_____
_____

To improve:

_____

When you want to give up, remember why you started

Six Month Review

Well done you have completed six months .

Physical Measurements:

Weight:	Change in weight:
Waist:	Change in waist:
Hips:	Change in hips:
Thigh:	Change in thigh:

Any other measurements:

	Change:
	Change:
	Change:
	Change:

Best thing about the last three months (since three month review):

What I need to improve:

Main goal for next three months:

Week Beginning: _____

Monday

🍎 Food:

_____
_____
_____
_____

Mood: 😄 😐 ☹️

✏️ Notes:

Water 💧
_____

Exercise 🏋️
_____

Sleep ⏱️

Tuesday

🍎 Food:

_____
_____
_____
_____

Mood: 😄 😐 ☹️

✏️ Notes:

Water 💧
_____

Exercise 🏋️
_____

Sleep ⏱️

Wednesday

🍎 Food:

_____
_____
_____
_____

Mood: 😄 😐 ☹️

✏️ Notes:

Water 💧
_____

Exercise 🏋️
_____

Sleep ⏱️

Thursday

🍎 Food:

_____
_____
_____
_____

Mood: 😄 😐 ☹️

✏️ Notes:

Water 💧
_____

Exercise 🏋️
_____

Sleep ⏱️

"Imagine yourself six months from now."

Friday

🍎 Food:

_____
_____
_____
_____

Mood: 😄 😐 ☹️

✏️ Notes:

Water 💧
_____

Exercise 🏋️
_____

Sleep ⏱️
_____

Saturday

🍎 Food:

_____
_____
_____
_____

Mood: 😄 😐 ☹️

✏️ Notes:

Water 💧
_____

Exercise 🏋️
_____

Sleep ⏱️
_____

Sunday

🍎 Food:

_____
_____
_____
_____

Mood: 😄 😐 ☹️

✏️ Notes:

Water 💧
_____

Exercise 🏋️
_____

Sleep ⏱️
_____

Week Overview

General mood: 😄 😐 ☹️

⚖️ Weight: _____

▭ Waist: _____

What went well:
....
....

To improve:
....
....

Week Beginning: _____

Monday

🍎 Food:

_____
_____
_____
_____

Mood: 😄 😐 ☹️   Water 💧

✏️ Notes: _____

                          Exercise 🏋️

                          _____

                          Sleep ⏱️

Tuesday

🍎 Food:

_____
_____
_____
_____

Mood: 😄 😐 ☹️   Water 💧

✏️ Notes: _____

                          Exercise 🏋️

                          _____

                          Sleep ⏱️

Wednesday

🍎 Food:

_____
_____
_____
_____

Mood: 😄 😐 ☹️   Water 💧

✏️ Notes: _____

                          Exercise 🏋️

                          _____

                          Sleep ⏱️

Thursday

🍎 Food:

_____
_____
_____
_____

Mood: 😄 😐 ☹️   Water 💧

✏️ Notes: _____

                          Exercise 🏋️

                          _____

                          Sleep ⏱️

"Imagine your life is perfect in every respect; what would it look like?" **Brian Tracy**

Friday

🍎 Food:

_____

_____

_____

_____

✏️ Mood: 😄 😐 ☹️

✏️ Notes:

Water 💧

_____

Exercise 🏋️

_____

Sleep ⏱️

_____

Saturday

🍎 Food:

_____

_____

_____

_____

Mood: 😄 😐 ☹️

✏️ Notes:

Water 💧

_____

Exercise 🏋️

_____

Sleep ⏱️

_____

Sunday

🍎 Food:

_____

_____

_____

_____

Mood: 😄 😐 ☹️

✏️ Notes:

Water 💧

_____

Exercise 🏋️

_____

Sleep ⏱️

_____

Week Overview

General mood: 😄 😐 ☹️

⚖️ Weight: _____

➖ Waist: _____

What went well:

_____

_____

To improve:

_____

Week Beginning: _____

Monday

🍎 Food:

_____

_____

_____

_____

Mood: 😄 😐 ☹️

✏️ Notes:

Water 💧
_____

Exercise 🏋️
_____

Sleep ⏱️

Tuesday

🍎 Food:

_____

_____

_____

_____

Mood: 😄 😐 ☹️

✏️ Notes:

Water 💧
_____

Exercise 🏋️
_____

Sleep ⏱️

Wednesday

🍎 Food:

_____

_____

_____

_____

Mood: 😄 😐 ☹️

✏️ Notes:

Water 💧
_____

Exercise 🏋️
_____

Sleep ⏱️

Thursday

🍎 Food:

_____

_____

_____

_____

Mood: 😄 😐 ☹️

✏️ Notes:

Water 💧
_____

Exercise 🏋️
_____

Sleep ⏱️

"Pain is temporary. Quitting lasts forever." Lance Armstrong

Friday

🍎 Food:

_____
_____
_____
_____

Mood: 😄 😐 ☹️   Water 💧
✏️ Notes:
_____
Exercise 🏋️
_____
Sleep ⏱️
_____

Saturday

🍎 Food:

_____
_____
_____
_____

Mood: 😄 😐 ☹️   Water 💧
✏️ Notes:
_____
Exercise 🏋️
_____
Sleep ⏱️
_____

Sunday

🍎 Food:

_____
_____
_____
_____

Mood: 😄 😐 ☹️   Water 💧
✏️ Notes:
_____
Exercise 🏋️
_____
Sleep ⏱️
_____

Week Overview

General mood: 😄 😐 ☹️

⚖️ Weight: _____

➖ Waist: _____

What went well:

_____
_____

To improve:

_____

Week Beginning: _____

Monday

🍎 Food:

_____
_____
_____

Mood: 😄 😐 ☹️   Water 💧

✏️ Notes: _____

Exercise 🏋️

_____

Sleep ⏱️

_____

Tuesday

🍎 Food:

_____
_____
_____

Mood: 😄 😐 ☹️   Water 💧

✏️ Notes: _____

Exercise 🏋️

_____

Sleep ⏱️

_____

Wednesday

🍎 Food:

_____
_____
_____

Mood: 😄 😐 ☹️   Water 💧

✏️ Notes: _____

Exercise 🏋️

_____

Sleep ⏱️

_____

Thursday

🍎 Food:

_____
_____
_____

Mood: 😄 😐 ☹️   Water 💧

✏️ Notes: _____

Exercise 🏋️

_____

Sleep ⏱️

_____

"A problem is a chance for you to do your best." Duke Ellington

Friday

🍎 Food:

_____
_____
_____
_____

Mood: 😄 😐 ☹️

Notes:

Water 💧
_____

Exercise 🏋️
_____

Sleep ⏱️
_____

Saturday

🍎 Food:

_____
_____
_____
_____

Mood: 😄 😐 ☹️

Notes:

Water 💧
_____

Exercise 🏋️
_____

Sleep ⏱️
_____

Sunday

🍎 Food:

_____
_____
_____
_____

Mood: 😄 😐 ☹️

Notes:

Water 💧
_____

Exercise 🏋️
_____

Sleep ⏱️
_____

Week Overview

General mood: 😄 😐 ☹️

⚖️ Weight: _____

➖ Waist: _____

What went well:

_____
_____

To improve:

_____

Week Beginning: _____

Monday

🍎 Food:

_____

_____

_____

_____

Mood: 😄 😐 ☹️

✏️ Notes:

Water 💧 _____

Exercise 🏋️ _____

Sleep ⏱️ _____

Tuesday

🍎 Food:

_____

_____

_____

_____

Mood: 😄 😐 ☹️

✏️ Notes:

Water 💧 _____

Exercise 🏋️ _____

Sleep ⏱️ _____

Wednesday

🍎 Food:

_____

_____

_____

_____

Mood: 😄 😐 ☹️

✏️ Notes:

Water 💧 _____

Exercise 🏋️ _____

Sleep ⏱️ _____

Thursday

🍎 Food:

_____

_____

_____

_____

Mood: 😄 😐 ☹️

✏️ Notes:

Water 💧 _____

Exercise 🏋️ _____

Sleep ⏱️ _____

*"Exercising should be about rewarding the body with endorphins and strength.
Not about punishing your body for what you've eaten."*

Friday

🍎 Food:

_____
_____
_____
_____

Mood: 😄 😐 ☹️

✏️ Notes:

Water 💧
_____

Exercise 🏋️
_____

Sleep ⏱️
_____

Saturday

🍎 Food:

_____
_____
_____
_____

Mood: 😄 😐 ☹️

✏️ Notes:

Water 💧
_____

Exercise 🏋️
_____

Sleep ⏱️
_____

Sunday

🍎 Food:

_____
_____
_____
_____

Mood: 😄 😐 ☹️

✏️ Notes:

Water 💧
_____

Exercise 🏋️
_____

Sleep ⏱️
_____

Week Overview

General mood: 😄 😐 ☹️

⚖️ Weight: _____

▭ Waist: _____

What went well:

_____

_____

To improve:

_____

_____

Week Beginning: _____

Monday

🍎 Food:

_____
_____
_____
_____

Mood: 😄 😐 ☹️   Water 💧
_____

✏️ Notes:

Exercise 🏋️
_____

Sleep ⏱️
_____

Tuesday

🍎 Food:

_____
_____
_____
_____

Mood: 😄 😐 ☹️   Water 💧
_____

✏️ Notes:

Exercise 🏋️
_____

Sleep ⏱️
_____

Wednesday

🍎 Food:

_____
_____
_____
_____

Mood: 😄 😐 ☹️   Water 💧
_____

✏️ Notes:

Exercise 🏋️
_____

Sleep ⏱️
_____

Thursday

🍎 Food:

_____
_____
_____
_____

Mood: 😄 😐 ☹️   Water 💧
_____

✏️ Notes:

Exercise 🏋️
_____

Sleep ⏱️
_____

"Motivation is something that has to come from within. Someone can help you light the fire. But you've got to keep it burning." Cassey Ho

Friday

🍎 Food:

_____
_____
_____
_____

Mood: 😄 😐 ☹️

✏️ Notes:

Water 💧
_____

Exercise 🏋️
_____

Sleep ⏱️
_____

Saturday

🍎 Food:

_____
_____
_____
_____

Mood: 😄 😐 ☹️

✏️ Notes:

Water 💧
_____

Exercise 🏋️
_____

Sleep ⏱️
_____

Sunday

🍎 Food:

_____
_____
_____
_____

Mood: 😄 😐 ☹️

✏️ Notes:

Water 💧
_____

Exercise 🏋️
_____

Sleep ⏱️
_____

Week Overview

General mood: 😄 😐 ☹️

⚖️ Weight: _____

➖ Waist: _____

What went well:

_____
_____

To improve:

_____

Week Beginning: _____

Monday

🍎 Food:
_____
_____
_____
_____

Mood: 😄 😐 ☹️

✎ Notes:

Water 💧
_____

Exercise 🏋️
_____

Sleep ⏱️
_____

Tuesday

🍎 Food:
_____
_____
_____
_____

Mood: 😄 😐 ☹️

✎ Notes:

Water 💧
_____

Exercise 🏋️
_____

Sleep ⏱️
_____

Wednesday

🍎 Food:
_____
_____
_____
_____

Mood: 😄 😐 ☹️

✎ Notes:

Water 💧
_____

Exercise 🏋️
_____

Sleep ⏱️
_____

Thursday

🍎 Food:
_____
_____
_____

Mood: 😄 😐 ☹️

✎ Notes:

Water 💧
_____

Exercise 🏋️
_____

Sleep ⏱️
_____

"Take it one day at a time. One step at a time."

Friday

🍎 Food:

_____

_____

_____

_____

Mood: 😄 😐 ☹️

✏️ Notes:

Water 💧

_____

Exercise 🏋️

_____

Sleep ⏱️

_____

Saturday

🍎 Food:

_____

_____

_____

_____

Mood: 😄 😐 ☹️

✏️ Notes:

Water 💧

_____

Exercise 🏋️

_____

Sleep ⏱️

_____

Sunday

🍎 Food:

_____

_____

_____

_____

Mood: 😄 😐 ☹️

✏️ Notes:

Water 💧

_____

Exercise 🏋️

_____

Sleep ⏱️

_____

Week Overview

General mood: 😄 😐 ☹️

⚖️ Weight: _____

▬ Waist: _____

What went well:

_____

_____

To improve:

_____

_____

Week Beginning: _____

Monday

🍎 Food:
_____
_____
_____
_____

Mood: 😄 😐 ☹️   Water 💧 _____

✏️ Notes: Exercise 🏋️ _____

Sleep ⏱️ _____

Tuesday

🍎 Food:
_____
_____
_____
_____

Mood: 😄 😐 ☹️   Water 💧 _____

✏️ Notes: Exercise 🏋️ _____

Sleep ⏱️ _____

Wednesday

🍎 Food:
_____
_____
_____
_____

Mood: 😄 😐 ☹️   Water 💧 _____

✏️ Notes: Exercise 🏋️ _____

Sleep ⏱️ _____

Thursday

🍎 Food:
_____
_____
_____
_____

Mood: 😄 😐 ☹️   Water 💧 _____

✏️ Notes: Exercise 🏋️ _____

Sleep ⏱️ _____

"Most people have no idea how good their body is designed to feel."   Kevin Trudeau

Friday

🍎 Food:

_____

_____

_____

_____

Mood: 😄 😐 ☹️

✏️ Notes:

Water 💧

_____

Exercise 🏋️

_____

Sleep ⏱️

_____

Saturday

🍎 Food:

_____

_____

_____

_____

Mood: 😄 😐 ☹️

✏️ Notes:

Water 💧

_____

Exercise 🏋️

_____

Sleep ⏱️

_____

Sunday

🍎 Food:

_____

_____

_____

_____

Mood: 😄 😐 ☹️

✏️ Notes:

Water 💧

_____

Exercise 🏋️

_____

Sleep ⏱️

_____

Week Overview

General mood: 😄 😐 ☹️

⚖️ Weight: _____

➖ Waist: _____

What went well:

_____

_____

To improve:

_____

Week Beginning: _____

Monday

🍎 Food:

_____

_____

_____

Mood: 😄 😐 ☹️   Water 💧

✏️ Notes: _____

Exercise 🏋️   _____

Sleep ⏱️   _____

Tuesday

🍎 Food:

_____

_____

_____

Mood: 😄 😐 ☹️   Water 💧

✏️ Notes: _____

Exercise 🏋️   _____

Sleep ⏱️   _____

Wednesday

🍎 Food:

_____

_____

_____

Mood: 😄 😐 ☹️   Water 💧

✏️ Notes: _____

Exercise 🏋️   _____

Sleep ⏱️   _____

Thursday

🍎 Food:

_____

_____

_____

Mood: 😄 😐 ☹️   Water 💧

✏️ Notes: _____

Exercise 🏋️   _____

Sleep ⏱️   _____

"Whether You Think You Can Or Think You Can't, You're Right." **Henry Ford**

Friday

🍎 Food:

_____

_____

_____

_____

Mood: 😄 😐 ☹️

✒️ Notes:

Water 💧

_____

Exercise 🏋️

_____

Sleep ⏱️

_____

Saturday

🍎 Food:

_____

_____

_____

_____

Mood: 😄 😐 ☹️

✒️ Notes:

Water 💧

_____

Exercise 🏋️

_____

Sleep ⏱️

_____

Sunday

🍎 Food:

_____

_____

_____

_____

Mood: 😄 😐 ☹️

✒️ Notes:

Water 💧

_____

Exercise 🏋️

_____

Sleep ⏱️

_____

Week Overview

General mood: 😄 😐 ☹️

⚖️ Weight: _____

➖ Waist: _____

What went well:

_____

_____

To improve:

_____

_____

Week Beginning: _____

Monday

🍎 Food:

_____
_____
_____
_____

Mood: 😄 😐 ☹️ Water 💧

✎ Notes:

Exercise 🏋️

Sleep ⏱️

Tuesday

🍎 Food:

_____
_____
_____
_____

Mood: 😄 😐 ☹️ Water 💧

✎ Notes:

Exercise 🏋️

Sleep ⏱️

Wednesday

🍎 Food:

_____
_____
_____
_____

Mood: 😄 😐 ☹️ Water 💧

✎ Notes:

Exercise 🏋️

Sleep ⏱️

Thursday

🍎 Food:

_____
_____
_____
_____

Mood: 😄 😐 ☹️ Water 💧

✎ Notes:

Exercise 🏋️

Sleep ⏱️

"It's not about perfect. It's about effort." Jillian Michaels

Friday

🍎 Food:

_____
_____
_____
_____

Mood: 😄 😐 ☹️

✏️ Notes:

Water 💧
_____

Exercise 🏋️
_____

Sleep ⏱️
_____

Saturday

🍎 Food:

_____
_____
_____
_____

Mood: 😄 😐 ☹️

✏️ Notes:

Water 💧
_____

Exercise 🏋️
_____

Sleep ⏱️
_____

Sunday

🍎 Food:

_____
_____
_____
_____

Mood: 😄 😐 ☹️

✏️ Notes:

Water 💧
_____

Exercise 🏋️
_____

Sleep ⏱️
_____

Week Overview

General mood: 😄 😐 ☹️

⚖️ Weight: _____

➖ Waist: _____

What went well:

_____
_____

To improve:

_____

Week Beginning: _____

Monday

🍎 Food:

_____

_____

_____

_____

Mood: 😄 😐 ☹️   Water 💧

_____

✏️ Notes:

Exercise 🏋️

_____

Sleep ⏱️

_____

Tuesday

🍎 Food:

_____

_____

_____

_____

Mood: 😄 😐 ☹️   Water 💧

_____

✏️ Notes:

Exercise 🏋️

_____

Sleep ⏱️

_____

Wednesday

🍎 Food:

_____

_____

_____

_____

Mood: 😄 😐 ☹️   Water 💧

_____

✏️ Notes:

Exercise 🏋️

_____

Sleep ⏱️

_____

Thursday

🍎 Food:

_____

_____

_____

_____

Mood: 😄 😐 ☹️   Water 💧

_____

✏️ Notes:

Exercise 🏋️

_____

Sleep ⏱️

_____

"Believe you can and you're halfway there." **Theodore Roosevelt**

Friday

🍎 Food:

_____
_____
_____
_____

Mood: 😄 😐 ☹️

✏️ Notes:

Water 💧
_____

Exercise 🏋️
_____

Sleep ⏱️
_____

Saturday

🍎 Food:

_____
_____
_____
_____

Mood: 😄 😐 ☹️

✏️ Notes:

Water 💧
_____

Exercise 🏋️
_____

Sleep ⏱️
_____

Sunday

🍎 Food:

_____
_____
_____
_____

Mood: 😄 😐 ☹️

✏️ Notes:

Water 💧
_____

Exercise 🏋️
_____

Sleep ⏱️
_____

Week Overview

General mood: 😄 😐 ☹️

⚖️ Weight: _____

➖ Waist: _____

What went well:

_____
_____

To improve:

_____

Week Beginning: _____

Monday

🍎 Food:

_____

_____

_____

Mood: 😄 😐 ☹️

✏️ Notes:

Water 💧

_____

Exercise 🏋️

_____

Sleep ⏱️

_____

Tuesday

🍎 Food:

_____

_____

_____

Mood: 😄 😐 ☹️

✏️ Notes:

Water 💧

_____

Exercise 🏋️

_____

Sleep ⏱️

_____

Wednesday

🍎 Food:

_____

_____

_____

Mood: 😄 😐 ☹️

✏️ Notes:

Water 💧

_____

Exercise 🏋️

_____

Sleep ⏱️

_____

Thursday

🍎 Food:

_____

_____

_____

Mood: 😄 😐 ☹️

✏️ Notes:

Water 💧

_____

Exercise 🏋️

_____

Sleep ⏱️

_____

"You are so much more than what you are going through." John Tew

Friday

🍎 Food:

_____
_____
_____
_____

Mood: 😄 😐 🙁

✏️ Notes:

Water 💧
_____

Exercise 🏋️
_____

Sleep ⏱️
_____

Saturday

🍎 Food:

_____
_____
_____
_____

Mood: 😄 😐 🙁

✏️ Notes:

Water 💧
_____

Exercise 🏋️
_____

Sleep ⏱️
_____

Sunday

🍎 Food:

_____
_____
_____
_____

Mood: 😄 😐 🙁

✏️ Notes:

Water 💧
_____

Exercise 🏋️
_____

Sleep ⏱️
_____

Week Overview

General mood: 😄 😐 🙁

⚖️ Weight: _____

➖ Waist: _____

What went well:

_____
_____

To improve:

_____

Week Beginning: _____

Monday

🍎 Food:

_____
_____
_____

Mood: 😄 😐 ☹️

✎ Notes:

Water 💧
_____
Exercise 🏋️
_____
Sleep ⏱️
_____

Tuesday

🍎 Food:

_____
_____
_____

Mood: 😄 😐 ☹️

✎ Notes:

Water 💧
_____
Exercise 🏋️
_____
Sleep ⏱️
_____

Wednesday

🍎 Food:

_____
_____
_____

Mood: 😄 😐 ☹️

✎ Notes:

Water 💧
_____
Exercise 🏋️
_____
Sleep ⏱️
_____

Thursday

🍎 Food:

_____
_____
_____

Mood: 😄 😐 ☹️

✎ Notes:

Water 💧
_____
Exercise 🏋️
_____
Sleep ⏱️
_____

"Difficult roads always lead to beautiful destinations." Zig Ziglar

Friday

🍎 Food:

_____
_____
_____
_____

Mood: 😄 😐 ☹️

✏️ Notes:

Water 💧
_____

Exercise 🏋️
_____

Sleep ⏱️
_____

Saturday

🍎 Food:

_____
_____
_____
_____

Mood: 😄 😐 ☹️

✏️ Notes:

Water 💧
_____

Exercise 🏋️
_____

Sleep ⏱️
_____

Sunday

🍎 Food:

_____
_____
_____
_____

Mood: 😄 😐 ☹️

✏️ Notes:

Water 💧
_____

Exercise 🏋️
_____

Sleep ⏱️
_____

Week Overview

General mood: 😄 😐 ☹️

⚖️ Weight: _____

▬ Waist: _____

What went well:

_____
_____

To improve:

_____
_____

Food is fuel
not therapy.

Three Monthly Review

Well done you have completed nine months.

Physical Measurements:

Weight:	Change in weight:
Waist:	Change in waist:
Hips:	Change in hips:
Thigh:	Change in thigh:

Any other measurements:

	Change:
	Change:
	Change:
	Change:

Best thing about the last three months:

What I need to improve:

Main goal for next three months:

Week Beginning: _____

Monday

🍎 Food:
_____
_____
_____
_____

Mood: 😄 😐 ☹️

✏️ Notes:

Water 💧
_____
Exercise 🏋️
_____
Sleep ⏱️
_____

Tuesday

🍎 Food:
_____
_____
_____
_____

Mood: 😄 😐 ☹️

✏️ Notes:

Water 💧
_____
Exercise 🏋️
_____
Sleep ⏱️
_____

Wednesday

🍎 Food:
_____
_____
_____
_____

Mood: 😄 😐 ☹️

✏️ Notes:

Water 💧
_____
Exercise 🏋️
_____
Sleep ⏱️
_____

Thursday

🍎 Food:
_____
_____
_____
_____

Mood: 😄 😐 ☹️

✏️ Notes:

Water 💧
_____
Exercise 🏋️
_____
Sleep ⏱️
_____

"Knowing is not enough; we must apply. Wishing is not enough; we must do."
Johann Wolfgang Von Goethe

Friday

🍎 Food:
_____
_____
_____
_____

Mood: 😄 😐 ☹️

✏️ Notes:

Water 💧
_____

Exercise 🏋️
_____

Sleep ⏱️
_____

Saturday

🍎 Food:
_____
_____
_____
_____

Mood: 😄 😐 ☹️

✏️ Notes:

Water 💧
_____

Exercise 🏋️
_____

Sleep ⏱️
_____

Sunday

🍎 Food:
_____
_____
_____
_____

Mood: 😄 😐 ☹️

✏️ Notes:

Water 💧
_____

Exercise 🏋️
_____

Sleep ⏱️
_____

Week Overview

General mood: 😄 😐 ☹️

⚖️ Weight: _____

➖ Waist: _____

What went well:
_____
_____

To improve:
_____
_____

Week Beginning: _____

Monday

🍎 Food:

_____
_____
_____

Mood: 😄 😐 🙁   Water 💧
_____

✏️ Notes: Exercise 🏋️
_____

Sleep ⏱️
_____

Tuesday

🍎 Food:

_____
_____
_____

Mood: 😄 😐 🙁   Water 💧
_____

✏️ Notes: Exercise 🏋️
_____

Sleep ⏱️
_____

Wednesday

🍎 Food:

_____
_____
_____

Mood: 😄 😐 🙁   Water 💧
_____

✏️ Notes: Exercise 🏋️
_____

Sleep ⏱️
_____

Thursday

🍎 Food:

_____
_____
_____

Mood: 😄 😐 🙁   Water 💧
_____

✏️ Notes: Exercise 🏋️
_____

Sleep ⏱️
_____

"If you keep going you won't regret it. If you give up you will."

Friday

🍎 Food:

_____

_____

_____

_____

Mood: 😄 😐 ☹️

✏️ Notes:

Water 💧
_____

Exercise 🏋️
_____

Sleep ⏱️
_____

Saturday

🍎 Food:

_____

_____

_____

_____

Mood: 😄 😐 ☹️

✏️ Notes:

Water 💧
_____

Exercise 🏋️
_____

Sleep ⏱️
_____

Sunday

🍎 Food:

_____

_____

_____

_____

Mood: 😄 😐 ☹️

✏️ Notes:

Water 💧
_____

Exercise 🏋️
_____

Sleep ⏱️
_____

Week Overview

General mood: 😄 😐 ☹️

⚖️ Weight: _____

➖ Waist: _____

What went well:

_____

_____

To improve:

_____

_____

Week Beginning: _____

Monday

🍎 Food:

_____

_____

_____

Mood: 😄 😐 ☹️

✏️ Notes:

Water 💧

_____

Exercise 🏋️

_____

Sleep ⏱️

Tuesday

🍎 Food:

_____

_____

_____

Mood: 😄 😐 ☹️

✏️ Notes:

Water 💧

_____

Exercise 🏋️

_____

Sleep ⏱️

Wednesday

🍎 Food:

_____

_____

_____

Mood: 😄 😐 ☹️

✏️ Notes:

Water 💧

_____

Exercise 🏋️

_____

Sleep ⏱️

Thursday

🍎 Food:

_____

_____

_____

Mood: 😄 😐 ☹️

✏️ Notes:

Water 💧

_____

Exercise 🏋️

_____

Sleep ⏱️

"Being challenged in life is inevitable. Being defeated is optional."

Friday

🍎 Food:

_____
_____
_____
_____

Mood: 😄 😐 ☹️

✒️ Notes:

Water 💧
_____

Exercise 🏋️
_____

Sleep ⏱️
_____

Saturday

🍎 Food:

_____
_____
_____
_____

Mood: 😄 😐 ☹️

✒️ Notes:

Water 💧
_____

Exercise 🏋️
_____

Sleep ⏱️
_____

Sunday

🍎 Food:

_____
_____
_____
_____

Mood: 😄 😐 ☹️

✒️ Notes:

Water 💧
_____

Exercise 🏋️
_____

Sleep ⏱️
_____

Week Overview

General mood: 😄 😐 ☹️

⚖️ Weight: _____

▬ Waist: _____

What went well:

_____
_____

To improve:

_____

Week Beginning: _____

Monday

🍎 Food:

_____
_____
_____
_____

Mood: 😄 😐 ☹️   Water 💧
_____
✏️ Notes: Exercise 🏋️
_____
Sleep ⏱️
_____

Tuesday

🍎 Food:

_____
_____
_____
_____

Mood: 😄 😐 ☹️   Water 💧
_____
✏️ Notes: Exercise 🏋️
_____
Sleep ⏱️
_____

Wednesday

🍎 Food:

_____
_____
_____
_____

Mood: 😄 😐 ☹️   Water 💧
_____
✏️ Notes: Exercise 🏋️
_____
Sleep ⏱️
_____

Thursday

🍎 Food:

_____
_____
_____
_____

Mood: 😄 😐 ☹️   Water 💧
_____
✏️ Notes: Exercise 🏋️
_____
Sleep ⏱️
_____

"And Yes, it is possible, and No, it isn't easy."

Friday

🍎 Food:

_____
_____
_____
_____

Mood: 😄 😐 ☹️

✏️ Notes:

Water 💧
_____

Exercise 🏋️
_____

Sleep ⏱️
_____

Saturday

🍎 Food:

_____
_____
_____
_____

Mood: 😄 😐 ☹️

✏️ Notes:

Water 💧
_____

Exercise 🏋️
_____

Sleep ⏱️
_____

Sunday

🍎 Food:

_____
_____
_____
_____

Mood: 😄 😐 ☹️

✏️ Notes:

Water 💧
_____

Exercise 🏋️
_____

Sleep ⏱️
_____

Week Overview

General mood: 😄 😐 ☹️

⚖️ Weight: _____

➖ Waist: _____

What went well:

_____
_____

To improve:

_____

Week Beginning: _____

Monday

🍎 Food:

_____
_____
_____
_____

Mood: 😄 😐 ☹️   Water 💧 _____

✏️ Notes:

Exercise 🏋️ _____

Sleep ⏱️ _____

Tuesday

🍎 Food:

_____
_____
_____
_____

Mood: 😄 😐 ☹️   Water 💧 _____

✏️ Notes:

Exercise 🏋️ _____

Sleep ⏱️ _____

Wednesday

🍎 Food:

_____
_____
_____
_____

Mood: 😄 😐 ☹️   Water 💧 _____

✏️ Notes:

Exercise 🏋️ _____

Sleep ⏱️ _____

Thursday

🍎 Food:

_____
_____
_____
_____

Mood: 😄 😐 ☹️   Water 💧 _____

✏️ Notes:

Exercise 🏋️ _____

Sleep ⏱️ _____

"Be stronger than your excuses."

Friday

🍎 Food:

_____
_____
_____
_____

Mood: 😄 😐 ☹️

✏️ Notes:

Water 💧
_____

Exercise 🏋️
_____

Sleep ⏱️
_____

Saturday

🍎 Food:

_____
_____
_____
_____

Mood: 😄 😐 ☹️

✏️ Notes:

Water 💧
_____

Exercise 🏋️
_____

Sleep ⏱️
_____

Sunday

🍎 Food:

_____
_____
_____
_____

Mood: 😄 😐 ☹️

✏️ Notes:

Water 💧
_____

Exercise 🏋️
_____

Sleep ⏱️
_____

Week Overview

General mood: 😄 😐 ☹️

⚖️ Weight: _____

▬ Waist: _____

What went well:

....
....

To improve:

....
....

Week Beginning: _____

Monday

🍎 Food:

_____
_____
_____
_____

Mood: 😄 😐 ☹️

✏️ Notes:

Water 💧
_____
Exercise 🏋️
_____
Sleep ⏱️
_____

Tuesday

🍎 Food:

_____
_____
_____
_____

Mood: 😄 😐 ☹️

✏️ Notes:

Water 💧
_____
Exercise 🏋️
_____
Sleep ⏱️
_____

Wednesday

🍎 Food:

_____
_____
_____
_____

Mood: 😄 😐 ☹️

✏️ Notes:

Water 💧
_____
Exercise 🏋️
_____
Sleep ⏱️
_____

Thursday

🍎 Food:

_____
_____
_____
_____

Mood: 😄 😐 ☹️

✏️ Notes:

Water 💧
_____
Exercise 🏋️
_____
Sleep ⏱️
_____

"The only person you should compare yourself to, is you yesterday."

Friday

🍎 Food:

_____
_____
_____
_____

Mood: 😄 😐 ☹️

✏️ Notes:

Water 💧
_____

Exercise 🏋️
_____

Sleep ⏱️
_____

Saturday

🍎 Food:

_____
_____
_____
_____

Mood: 😄 😐 ☹️

✏️ Notes:

Water 💧
_____

Exercise 🏋️
_____

Sleep ⏱️
_____

Sunday

🍎 Food:

_____
_____
_____
_____

Mood: 😄 😐 ☹️

✏️ Notes:

Water 💧
_____

Exercise 🏋️
_____

Sleep ⏱️
_____

Week Overview

General mood: 😄 😐 ☹️

⚖️ Weight: _____

➖ Waist: _____

What went well:

_____
_____

To improve:

_____

Week Beginning: _____

Monday

🍎 Food:

_____

_____

_____

_____

Mood: 😄 😐 ☹️

✎ Notes:

Water 💧

_____

Exercise 🏋️

_____

Sleep ⏱️

_____

Tuesday

🍎 Food:

_____

_____

_____

_____

Mood: 😄 😐 ☹️

✎ Notes:

Water 💧

_____

Exercise 🏋️

_____

Sleep ⏱️

_____

Wednesday

🍎 Food:

_____

_____

_____

_____

Mood: 😄 😐 ☹️

✎ Notes:

Water 💧

_____

Exercise 🏋️

_____

Sleep ⏱️

_____

Thursday

🍎 Food:

_____

_____

_____

_____

Mood: 😄 😐 ☹️

✎ Notes:

Water 💧

_____

Exercise 🏋️

_____

Sleep ⏱️

_____

"You get what you work for, not what you wish for."

Friday

Food:

_____

_____

_____

_____

Mood: 😄 😐 ☹️

Notes:

Water 💧

_____

Exercise 🏋️

_____

Sleep ⏱️

_____

Saturday

Food:

_____

_____

_____

_____

Mood: 😄 😐 ☹️

Notes:

Water 💧

_____

Exercise 🏋️

_____

Sleep ⏱️

_____

Sunday

Food:

_____

_____

_____

_____

Mood: 😄 😐 ☹️

Notes:

Water 💧

_____

Exercise 🏋️

_____

Sleep ⏱️

_____

Week Overview

General mood: 😄 😐 ☹️

⚖️ Weight: _____

➖ Waist: _____

What went well:

_____

_____

To improve:

_____

Week Beginning: _____

Monday

🍎 Food:

_____

_____

_____

_____

Mood: 😄 😐 ☹️

✏️ Notes:

Water 💧
_____

Exercise 🏋️
_____

Sleep ⏱️
_____

Tuesday

🍎 Food:

_____

_____

_____

_____

Mood: 😄 😐 ☹️

✏️ Notes:

Water 💧
_____

Exercise 🏋️
_____

Sleep ⏱️
_____

Wednesday

🍎 Food:

_____

_____

_____

_____

Mood: 😄 😐 ☹️

✏️ Notes:

Water 💧
_____

Exercise 🏋️
_____

Sleep ⏱️
_____

Thursday

🍎 Food:

_____

_____

_____

_____

Mood: 😄 😐 ☹️

✏️ Notes:

Water 💧
_____

Exercise 🏋️
_____

Sleep ⏱️
_____

"It is your determination and persistence that will make you a successful person."
Kenneth J Hutchins

Friday

🍎 Food:

_____

_____

_____

_____

Mood: 😄 😐 ☹️

✒️ Notes:

Water 💧
_____

Exercise 🏋️
_____

Sleep ⏱️
_____

Saturday

🍎 Food:

_____

_____

_____

_____

Mood: 😄 😐 ☹️

✒️ Notes:

Water 💧
_____

Exercise 🏋️
_____

Sleep ⏱️
_____

Sunday

🍎 Food:

_____

_____

_____

_____

Mood: 😄 😐 ☹️

✒️ Notes:

Water 💧
_____

Exercise 🏋️
_____

Sleep ⏱️
_____

Week Overview

General mood: 😄 😐 ☹️

⚖️ Weight: _____

➖ Waist: _____

What went well:

_____

_____

To improve:

_____

Week Beginning: _____

Monday

🍎 Food:

_____
_____
_____
_____

Mood: 😄 😐 ☹️

✎ Notes:

Water 💧

_____

Exercise 🏋️

_____

Sleep ⏱️

_____

Tuesday

🍎 Food:

_____
_____
_____
_____

Mood: 😄 😐 ☹️

✎ Notes:

Water 💧

_____

Exercise 🏋️

_____

Sleep ⏱️

_____

Wednesday

🍎 Food:

_____
_____
_____
_____

Mood: 😄 😐 ☹️

✎ Notes:

Water 💧

_____

Exercise 🏋️

_____

Sleep ⏱️

_____

Thursday

🍎 Food:

_____
_____
_____
_____

Mood: 😄 😐 ☹️

✎ Notes:

Water 💧

_____

Exercise 🏋️

_____

Sleep ⏱️

_____

"#1 make good decisions, #2 everything else." **Rand Fishkin**

Friday

🍎 Food:

_____

_____

_____

_____

Mood: 😄 😐 ☹️

🖊 Notes:

Water 💧

_____

Exercise 🏋

_____

Sleep ⏱

_____

Saturday

🍎 Food:

_____

_____

_____

_____

Mood: 😄 😐 ☹️

🖊 Notes:

Water 💧

_____

Exercise 🏋

_____

Sleep ⏱

_____

Sunday

🍎 Food:

_____

_____

_____

_____

Mood: 😄 😐 ☹️

🖊 Notes:

Water 💧

_____

Exercise 🏋

_____

Sleep ⏱

_____

Week Overview

General mood: 😄 😐 ☹️

⚖ Weight: _____

➖ Waist: _____

What went well:

_____

_____

To improve:

_____

Week Beginning: _____

Monday

🍎 Food:

_____
_____
_____
_____

Mood: 😄 😐 ☹️   Water 💧

✏️ Notes:

Exercise 🏋️

Sleep ⏱️

Tuesday

🍎 Food:

_____
_____
_____
_____

Mood: 😄 😐 ☹️   Water 💧

✏️ Notes:

Exercise 🏋️

Sleep ⏱️

Wednesday

🍎 Food:

_____
_____
_____
_____

Mood: 😄 😐 ☹️   Water 💧

✏️ Notes:

Exercise 🏋️

Sleep ⏱️

Thursday

🍎 Food:

_____
_____
_____
_____

Mood: 😄 😐 ☹️   Water 💧

✏️ Notes:

Exercise 🏋️

Sleep ⏱️

"The number one reason people fail in life is because they listen to their friends, family, and neighbors." Napoleon Hill

Friday

🍎 Food:

_____
_____
_____
_____

Mood: 😄 😐 ☹️   Water 💧
_____

✏️ Notes: Exercise 🏋️
_____

Sleep ⏱️
_____

Saturday

🍎 Food:

_____
_____
_____
_____

Mood: 😄 😐 ☹️   Water 💧
_____

✏️ Notes: Exercise 🏋️
_____

Sleep ⏱️
_____

Sunday

🍎 Food:

_____
_____
_____
_____

Mood: 😄 😐 ☹️   Water 💧
_____

✏️ Notes: Exercise 🏋️
_____

Sleep ⏱️
_____

Week Overview

General mood: 😄 😐 ☹️

⚖️ Weight: _____

➖ Waist: _____

What went well:

_____
_____

To improve:

_____

Week Beginning: _____

Monday

🍎 Food:

_____
_____
_____

Mood: 😄 😐 ☹️   Water 💧 _____

✎ Notes:

Exercise 🏋️ _____

Sleep ⏱️ _____

Tuesday

🍎 Food:

_____
_____
_____

Mood: 😄 😐 ☹️   Water 💧 _____

✎ Notes:

Exercise 🏋️ _____

Sleep ⏱️ _____

Wednesday

🍎 Food:

_____
_____
_____

Mood: 😄 😐 ☹️   Water 💧 _____

✎ Notes:

Exercise 🏋️ _____

Sleep ⏱️ _____

Thursday

🍎 Food:

_____
_____
_____

Mood: 😄 😐 ☹️   Water 💧 _____

✎ Notes:

Exercise 🏋️ _____

Sleep ⏱️ _____

Every time you eat or drink you are either feeding disease or fighting it.

Friday

🍎 Food:

_____
_____
_____
_____

Mood: 😄 😐 ☹️

✏️ Notes:

Water 💧
_____

Exercise 🏋️
_____

Sleep ⏱️
_____

Saturday

🍎 Food:

_____
_____
_____
_____

Mood: 😄 😐 ☹️

✏️ Notes:

Water 💧
_____

Exercise 🏋️
_____

Sleep ⏱️
_____

Sunday

🍎 Food:

_____
_____
_____
_____

Mood: 😄 😐 ☹️

✏️ Notes:

Water 💧
_____

Exercise 🏋️
_____

Sleep ⏱️
_____

Week Overview

General mood: 😄 😐 ☹️

⚖️ Weight: _____

➖ Waist: _____

What went well:

_____

To improve:

_____

Week Beginning: _____

Monday

🍎 Food:
_____
_____
_____

Mood: 😄 😐 ☹️   Water 💧
✏️ Notes: _____
                   Exercise 🏋️
                   _____
                   Sleep ⏱️
                   _____

Tuesday

🍎 Food:
_____
_____
_____

Mood: 😄 😐 ☹️   Water 💧
✏️ Notes: _____
                   Exercise 🏋️
                   _____
                   Sleep ⏱️
                   _____

Wednesday

🍎 Food:
_____
_____
_____

Mood: 😄 😐 ☹️   Water 💧
✏️ Notes: _____
                   Exercise 🏋️
                   _____
                   Sleep ⏱️
                   _____

Thursday

🍎 Food:
_____
_____
_____

Mood: 😄 😐 ☹️   Water 💧
✏️ Notes: _____
                   Exercise 🏋️
                   _____
                   Sleep ⏱️
                   _____

*"Two roads diverged in a wood and I took the one less traveled by,
and that made all the difference."* Robert Frost

Friday

🍎 Food:

_____
_____
_____
_____

Mood: 😄 😐 ☹️

✏️ Notes:

Water 💧
_____

Exercise 🏋️
_____

Sleep ⏱️
_____

Saturday

🍎 Food:

_____
_____
_____
_____

Mood: 😄 😐 ☹️

✏️ Notes:

Water 💧
_____

Exercise 🏋️
_____

Sleep ⏱️
_____

Sunday

🍎 Food:

_____
_____
_____
_____

Mood: 😄 😐 ☹️

✏️ Notes:

Water 💧
_____

Exercise 🏋️
_____

Sleep ⏱️
_____

Week Overview

General mood: 😄 😐 ☹️

⚖️ Weight: _____

➖ Waist: _____

What went well:

_____
_____

To improve:

_____

Week Beginning: _____

Monday

🍎 Food:

_____

_____

_____

_____

Mood: 😄 😐 ☹️   Water 💧

✏️ Notes: _____

Exercise 🏋️ _____

Sleep ⏱️ _____

Tuesday

🍎 Food:

_____

_____

_____

_____

Mood: 😄 😐 ☹️   Water 💧

✏️ Notes: _____

Exercise 🏋️ _____

Sleep ⏱️ _____

Wednesday

🍎 Food:

_____

_____

_____

_____

Mood: 😄 😐 ☹️   Water 💧

✏️ Notes: _____

Exercise 🏋️ _____

Sleep ⏱️ _____

Thursday

🍎 Food:

_____

_____

_____

_____

Mood: 😄 😐 ☹️   Water 💧

✏️ Notes: _____

Exercise 🏋️ _____

Sleep ⏱️ _____

"Don't dig your grave with your own knife and fork." Old English Proverb

Friday

🍎 Food:

_____
_____
_____
_____

Mood: 😄 😐 ☹️   Water 💧
_____

✏️ Notes:

Exercise 🏋️
_____

Sleep ⏱️
_____

Saturday

🍎 Food:

_____
_____
_____
_____

Mood: 😄 😐 ☹️   Water 💧
_____

✏️ Notes:

Exercise 🏋️
_____

Sleep ⏱️
_____

Sunday

🍎 Food:

_____
_____
_____
_____

Mood: 😄 😐 ☹️   Water 💧
_____

✏️ Notes:

Exercise 🏋️
_____

Sleep ⏱️
_____

Week Overview

General mood: 😄 😐 ☹️

⚖️ Weight: _____

➖ Waist: _____

What went well:

_____
_____

To improve:

_____

Annual Review

Well done you have completed a year.

Physical Measurements:

Weight:	Change in weight:
Waist:	Change in waist:
Hips:	Change in hips:
Thigh:	Change in thigh:

Any other measurements:

	Change:
	Change:
	Change:
	Change:

Best thing about the last year:

What I need to improve:

Main goal for next year:

Being on a healthy diet is not about feeling hungry and deprived. It is about nourishing yourself with whole foods, so you feel satisfied, energised and able to live life to the fullest.

www.ingramcontent.com/pod-product-compliance
Lightning Source LLC
Chambersburg PA
CBHW080559030426
42336CB00019B/3255